CBD Oil and Hemp Oil

The Ultimate Beginners Guide to CBD-Rich Hemp Oil to reduce pains

Includes tips and tricks to buy high quality CBD Oil to get you back in the groove

Hirsch Friedrich Pebble

Dedication

I desire sincerely for those seeking an alternative solution to synthetic medications, that they may experience relief when using CBD products.

Table of Content

PAGE LEFT INTENTIONALLY

Introduction

This book is written to serve as a guide to help the user of CBD oil know the meaning of CBD oil and Hemp Oil and to know the differences between both.

This book will answer common questions related to using CBD Oil.

CBD Oil is an amazing food, cosmetic and medicinal product. The CBD oil is used in its pure form and in combination with other oils. It is well tolerable with other medicines and can be used to treat diseases independently.

The CBD restores and protects the skin. It removes inflammation, irritation and wrinkles.

This oil is quickly absorbed and it leaves no oily traces.

This book will answer common questions related to using CBD oil such as:

Is CBD oil legal to use?

Will CBD oil get me high?

Does using the CBD oil have side effects?

How much of CBD oil can I take?

Where do I buy the CBD oil?

How can I buy the CBD oil online?

What are the health benefits of CBD oil?

And much more!

The CBD oil is quickly becoming a popular alternative to taking drugs as more and more people have found it does work.

The CBD oil is mostly confused by many to mean marijuana but this book will get that notion out of your mind. This book explains the differences between CBD hemp oil and marijuana.

The oil contains essential vitamins, calcium, micro and macro elements, magnesium, as well as amino acids that are essential to the body.

The hemp seed oil is also used as spices for food and this book contains some meal preparation that can be spiced with the hemp seed.

Chapter 1

What Is Hemp Seed?

Hemp belongs to the collection of plant trees in the family of Cannabis. This useful and multipurpose plant is often used for cloth, fibres, fuel, oil, resin, wax, and a large range of different helpful products. Hemp grows everywhere around the globe. Hemp is a strong plant and grows in any type of environmental surroundings.

This plant has been prohibited by some countries to be used or grown because it is believed that they have THC, a psycho-tropic chemical, which some individuals use as narcotics. However, some major countries have fashioned out the kinds of hemp that does not have the elements of THC. Currently, a dialogue concerning the utilization of cannabis which is commonly referred to by all as "marijuana", is ongoing, for the treatment of a large number of health conditions and problems.

The Nutritional Facts of Hemp Seed

The Hemp seed is extensively used all over the globe due to its health benefits, availability, sustainability and versatility. What make the hemp seeds so valuable are largely its chemical constituents, minerals and nutrients. These chemical components include iron, calcium, and magnesium, high amount of zinc, fiber and phosphorus.

Asides this, hemp seed comprises of a whole twenty one amino acids together with the 9 important amino acids which makes the hemp seeds a whole protein. In addition to this, hemp seeds are made up of a wide variety of important fats found in the body system as well as a large number of edible oils in addition to its rare kind of polyunsaturated fatty acid referred to as Gamma Linoleic Acid (GLA).

Benefits of the Hemp Seed

Hemp seed is incredibly useful in treating several ailments. This is attributed to the variety of nutrients it contains. Below are the health benefits of the hemp seeds.

1. It improves the Cardiovascular Health

The hemp seed does a great good on the heart, together with the appropriate balance of fatty acid or cholesterol present inside the body. Many health specialists around the world recommend an exact ratio of three to one or four to one (3:1 or 4:1) polyunsaturated fatty acid carboxylic acid to omega-3 fatty acid. This is the only plant matter in the universe which has a normal balance itself.

Adequate equilibrium of saturated cholesterol (fats) within the body is important for the body to function in a normal way, and to also prevent certain conditions such as heart attacks, atherosclerosis and strokes.

Since hemp seed contains a high amount of fiber, there is a boost which enhances healthy heart since fiber scrapes out surplus fats from the artery wall which results in heart related conditions. It then transports them to the excretory system where they are worked on and eliminated.

In addition, hemp seed has an ultimate distinctive characteristic. The GLA, (Gamma Linoleic Acid), is a unique kind of omega-six fatty acid, found in only a small number of edible sources, although it has great influence on one's health.

Hemp seed is also associated with enhancing a number of cardiovascular ailments and it also help to reduce the cholesterol that is not useful, while it increases the useful cholesterol present in the body.

In all, hemp seed contains a powerful substance that prevents injury to one's heart.

2. It boosts the digestive Health

This seed is a tremendous source of nutritional fiber for both soluble and insoluble, in a quantitative ratio four to one.

The insoluble fiber bulks up stool and enables the passage of stool within the digestive canal, thereby decreasing symptoms of constipation and bowel disorder.

The soluble fiber is in charge of slowing down the rate of absorption of glucose and increases the gastric and digestive juices, which also eases the movement of bowels. This fiber stimulates bile juice; which is responsible for reducing the bad fats in the body.

In all, these two fibers in the body help to prevent a great number of health conditions including cardiovascular disease and colorectal cancer.

3. It relieves sleep disorder (Insomnia)

The major importance of hemp seed is the availability of its rich mineral content such as magnesium which produces a really soothing and restful sensation across the body. The magnesium mineral compound has stimulating values on hormones and enzymes that causes sleep.

Once magnesium is used, serotonin is secreted which travels to the brain, where it is converted to melatonin.

This melatonin supports sleep powerfully. Sufferers of insomnia often claims that magnesium intake causes sleep greatly.

Please note that a serving of this seed daily has about fifty percent of the recommended magnesium dose. So, if you desire a restorative sleep, get a handful of hemp seeds.

4. It prevents Osteoporosis

The hemp seed contains calcium, an important element in strengthening and creation of bones. It also repairs damaged bones. The calcium derived from the seeds and hemp seed oil helps to reduce the possibilities of developing medical disorders like osteoporosis.

5. Used in the treatment of Anaemia

Iron is another mineral found in hemp seed. It is an important mineral of the red blood production inside the human body. When Iron is deficient in the body, it results into anaemia. Thus, eating foods adequate in iron can prevent anaemia, which presents itself in signs like headaches, fatigue, weakness in muscles, and a variety of other symptoms.

6. Used for Weight Loss

Hemp seed can be consumed in large amount without the fear of adding excess weight because they are low in calories and sodium, and it is also a complete protein. Having complete proteins in the body makes the body to feel full as a result of the amino acids that have been consumed through eating, thus repressing the secretion of ghrelin and controlling pains felt as a result of hunger. This lowers the possibilities of eating excessively and gaining undue weight.

In addition, fiber intake fills the body, aids digestion and eases bowel passage. It reduces weight gain and increase the effective incorporation of nutrients.

7. It boosts the body muscle mass

The hemp seed is considered a complete protein because of the presence of the eight important amino acids which cannot be produced by the body. These amino acids are effective for creating new body tissues inside the body and for strengthening muscle density and muscle mass.

Eating the right quantity of hemp seed boosts the muscles.

8. It prevents cancer

The oil and seed of hemp contains a specific amount of phenolic compounds which acts as potent antioxidants for the prevention of various kinds of cancer by removing free radicals.

These free radicals are poisonous by-products of cellular metabolism, liable to cause harm to cells that are healthy by altering their DNA (deoxyribonucleic acid) into cancerous cells.

Taking certain food such as hemp seeds can boost the phenolic content in the body, thus preventing cancer cells from developing in the body.

9. It strengthens the Immune system

The body immune system is boosted when there are many nutrients, minerals, vitamins, phenolic compounds, varieties of beneficial oils, and fiber. The immune system defends the body system against any health sickness and diseases.

10. Regulation of hormonal Imbalance

Hemp seed contains linoleic acids. The linoleic acid regulates +the hormone for pancreas and thyroid, and also works well at reducing several symptoms that result from hormonal imbalance such as anxiety, depression, mood swings and severe menopausal symptoms.

Hemp seed also helps to control the hormones causing hunger and weight gain. In all, the human body will function at an ideal and optimal level if the hormones in the body are well balanced.

Skin Benefits of Hemp Seed Oil

Hemp seed oil has exceptionally nourishing oil for pores and skin. It penetrates your pores and skin, tightens and gives powerful antioxidant to help achieve a stunning skin.

Hemp seed oil is full of many components that essentially act as food on your pores and skin, leaving it healthy and well nourished. Listed below are the benefits of the hemp oil to the skin:

1. It plumps worn-out, dry skin: The oil rejuvenates the skin thereby creating a refreshing youthful glow.

2. Long lasting moisture: The oil provides long lasting moisture to skins that easily gets dried. If your skin gets dried during the day, the oil provides the extra moisture your body needs. The continuous use of the oil will cause the skin not to get dried again.

3. Balances oily skin: Hemp seed oil is often thought to be the essential skin moisturizer because it doesn't clog pores.

4. It releases the skin. Using the seed oil takes away every form of skin irritation. The essential moisture it provides calms and relaxes the skin.

5. Less appearance of fine lines and wrinkles: The oil guards against different environmental factors and it also helps to reduce fine lines and wrinkles on the face.

6. It can be used by all skin types: No matter the texture of your skin, the hemp seed oil works perfectly on any

type of skin. It gives a soothing effect and a calming

relief to all dried and oily skin.

Chapter 2

What Is CBD Oil?

CBD oil is a botanical oil produced from the seeds and stalks of the cannabis plants. These plants are naturally rich in CBD and contain a low THC. It has a specialised technique used to extract the CBD oil and it contains nutritious elements such as vitamins, terpenes, omega-three fatty acids, minerals, amino acids and chlorophyll.

The CBD hemp oil is seen in most health food stores and markets. The hemp oil is obtained from the hemp seed containing only trace volume of CBD. The products of hemp seed contains very low quantity of CBD with regards to weight which makes them insufficient for those who seek to balance the CBD effect.

The need for CBD hemp oil has increased in the recent years making the market to respond by coming up with new and different types of products of CBD oil. There are varieties of CBD hemp oil product in the market.

Natural and pure CBD oil that can be used on their own are now available in drops, tablets, tinctures, drinks, and chewing gum.

If you are one of those who avoid trace amounts of THC seen in almost all the products of CBD hemp oil, then, the no amount-THC of CBD hemp oil products are now available in many stores and markets recently.

Consequences of CBD Oil

Although CBD oil will not cause the user to feel "high", many consumers of the CBD oil as an alternative to medicine or a nutritional enhancement have attested to feel an intensified sensation after taking their daily dose of CBD oil.

As soon as the body takes in CBD, the compound networks with cannabinoid and non-cannabinoid receptors to promote stability in an extensive range of structures. Research has shown over the decade that CBD facilitates the system of endocannabinoid to keep the body in homeostasis. Research advocates that CBD's connects with the receptors of the endocannabinoid system to manage seizure activities, reduce anxiety, decrease infection, fight despair, and provide antioxidant and neuro-protective properties that could possibly help in treating cardiovascular disease, Parkinson's ailment, stroke, arthritis and Alzheimer's disease.

In all, CBD oil is regarded as safe and best tolerated in the body system. Aside from users who have reported feelings of drowsiness and dry mouth, CBD oil has not been described to cause any noteworthy negative consequence.

Will CBD Oil get me high?

The major question asked by users of cannabidiol (CBD) is about its compound properties and to know about the benefits of taking CBD oil. Users really want to know if taking or using the CBD oil will intoxicate them.

The shortest answer to this question is a capital NO! CBD oil cannot get any one high. CBD oil is hauled out from cannabis plant.

A common fallacy is that it will bring out a euphoric result, but the basic truth is that, CBD oil is absolutely non-psychoactive, and does not in any way have an adverse effect on attention, behaviour, perception or sensory cognizance.

CBD oil has no extra trace quantity of (THC) tetrahydrocannabinol, which happens to be the psychoactive cannabinoid that provokes the "dim" or "stoned" mind-changing feelings which might be generally related to the use of marijuana. CBD oil is taken out from the seeds and stalks of hemp that contains only about 0.3 percent of THC per dry weight, or thirty-three times lower than the least powerful euphoric-initiating cannabis strain.

Rather, the CBD oil contains a whole lot of CBD, which has proven to have the competence to counter the psychoactive properties of THC.

Chapter 3

Difference between Hemp Oil and CBD

There are few correlated questions of cannabis that generates lots of controversy and discussion as "What is the difference between hemp oil and CBD oil?" The misunderstanding of these two stems from the usage of the word "hemp" to mean the type of marijuana that is used for medicinal or recreational purposes.

As it has been discussed in previous chapters, CBD oil and hemp oil are widely two different cannabis products.

As you proceed in this study, you will get to know what distinguishes the hemp oil from CBD oil, and why the usage of the phrase "hemp" as an extensive term for marijuana product is incorrect. The focus shall be on five definite variations between CBD oil and hemp oil:

1.   Origin of the species

2.   Parts that produces the oil

3.   Cannabinoid content

4.   Production Method

5.   Uses

1) Hemp oil vs. CBD oil: Origin of the Species

Hemp oil and CBD oil may seem to be the same on the surface. This is due to the origin of the plant. They both come from the same plant species.

The cannabis plant belongs to the genus cannabis, hence the derivation of its name. Within that genus are three species:

1. Sativa

2. Indica

3. Ruderalis

Species from *Cannabis Indica, Cannabis sativa* and fusion of the two comprises the bulk of the products you can easily find at any local dispensary. *Cannabis ruderalis*, on the other hand grows inside the wild. Asides this, it naturally has a low concentration of THC.

Hemp oil and CBD oil are both from the plant *Cannabis sativa*, even though some researchers have proven that hemp is more genetically akin to *Cannabis Indica*.

Though hemp oil and CBD oil come from the same genus and species *(Cannabis sativa),* hemp oil is derived from a strain that has a very low cannabinoid count while CBD oil is derived from the strains you can find in your local dispensary.

2) Hemp Oil vs. CBD oil: Parts that produces the oil

Hemp Oil is produced from the seeds of the hemp plant, similar to oils derived from almonds, coconuts and olives. CBD oil is produced from the leaves, flowers, and stalks of the *Cannabis Sativa* plant.

This does not mean that the leaves, flowers and stalks of the hemp plant are useless. As shall be later discussed in subsequent chapters, it would be noted that all parts of the hemp plant is useful and can be used in one way or the other.

The major thing for you to know is that hemp is not medicinal or psychoactive like the *Cannabis sativa* plant. This is mainly because the hemp plant is extremely low in cannabinoids.

Meaning of Cannabinoids

Cannabinoids are chemical compounds that act on the cannabinoid receptors in the human brain. Cannabidiol (CBD) and Delta9-Tetrahydrocannbinol (THC) are the most common cannabinoids around. Others include:

1. Cannabidiolic acid (CBDA).

2. Tetrahydrocannabinolic acid (THCA).

3. Cannabigerol (CBG).

4. Cannabigerolic acid (CBGA).

5. Tetrahydrocannabivarin (THCV).

6. Cannabichromene (CBC).

7. Cannabichromenate (CBCA).

8. Cannabinol (CBN) and lots more.

There are over 115 different cannabinoids that contributes in one way or the other to the medical and psychoactive experience.

3. Hemp Oil vs. CBD Oil: Cannabinoid content

The growers of marijuana focus typically on the two main cannabinoids: CBD and THC. They cross strains pass to produce new variations that increase one cannabinoid whilst decreasing the other. Take for instance, CBD has been proven to be extraordinarily beneficial in treating many medical conditions. This has caused the growers to create strains with high CBD and low THC.

Hemp Oil and CBD Oil are both Low in THC

Both hemp oil and CBD oil are low in THC when compared to other marijuana products. Most countries require that, to be taken into consideration as hemp, the concentration of THC must be lower or equal to 0.3%. There is no way one can feel high on marijuana at such a low percentage.

CBD oil may have a higher THC count but the concentration is usually between 1% and 5%. To optimally maximize the medicinal effects of CBD, the strains used to produce the CBD oil is of great importance.

Hemp Oil has Low CBD

Hemp oil has an extremely low CBD count of 3.5%. This low concentration makes it all but useless as a medical remedy. Due to the low cannabinoid count (THC and CBD), the hemp plant and specifically the hemp oil has massively distinctive uses when compared to CBD oil.

CBD Oil Has High CBD

CBD oil has a very high CBD count of 20%. This excessive concentration makes it ideal as a medical treatment for ailments such as anxiety, nausea, depression, cancer and seizures.

4. Hemp Oil vs. CBD Oil: Uses

As stated earlier, hemp oil is used for different purposes than its counterpart, CBD oil.

Hemp Oil doubles as a foodstuff and Industrial Product

Hemp oil, just as coconut oil and olive oil, is primarily a foodstuff. It is high in:

1. Vitamin E

2. Vitamin B1

3. Vitamin B2

4. Magnesium

5. Polyunsaturated fats (omega-3 & omega-6).

6. Potassium.

Hemp oil is likewise used for numerous industrial purposes, such as in the production of creams, bio-diesel gasoline, plastics, paint, soaps and shampoo. While hemp can provide healthy diet benefits, it is nothing compared to the health benefits of CBD

Uses of CBD oil

CBD oil is a Medicine

CBD oil is a medicine used in treating many health conditions such as:

1. Nausea and vomiting.

2. Anxiety

3. Bone growth

4. Nervous system degeneration

5. Chronic pain

6. Cancer cell growth

7. Insomnia

8. Low appetite

9. Bacteria growth

10.High blood sugar

11.Muscle spasms

12.Artery blockage

13.Inflammation

14.Seizures and convulsions

15.Psychoses

16.Psoriasis

Hemp oil is not a Medicine

Hemp oil is not used for healing. This is the significant difference. This should be taken into consideration as you would not want to go up to the counter at your local dispensary to ask for hemp oil with the intent of relieving your anxiety.

5) Hemp Oil vs. CBD Oil: Production Method

Another difference between CBD oil and hemp oil is their respective method of production.

These production methods are:

i. Pressing: Hemp oil is produced by pressing the seeds of the hemp plant. The process of extracting the oil by pressing the hemp seeds is very much akin to the processes used in producing other known oil like sesame, olive, peanut, coconut, etc.

ii. Solvent Extraction: The CBD oil is produced through the technique known as solvent extraction. A solvent like butane, alcohol, or carbon dioxide is forced across and through the Cannabis sativa plant matter from where it separates the cannabinoids, trichomes, and terpenes. The solvent is then allowed to evaporate, leaving behind the cannabinoid-packed CBD oil.

Hemp Oil Extraction Technique

Many of reviews of the CBD oil I have come across reveals that many users of CBD want to know why the CBD oil is very costly. This question typically comes from individuals who come across hemp oil in dispensaries and supermarkets offered at reduced prices. Hemp oil extraction is an important element to be considered.

The answer to that question is that CBD is different from the hemp seed oil. The technique of extraction for producing the rich cannabinoid products are not the same as those used for getting oil from hemp seed.

Hemp seed oil is manufactured by cold pressing the seeds and then removing the oil. This method is very easy to carry out in the house because it needs no special solvent or equipment. However, it must be noted that this oil which has nutritional value is not the same as the health-improving supplement produced. With this, we shall look into the different methods of hemp oil extraction.

1. Cold pressing as hemp oil extraction method.

Hemp seed oil is extremely rich in nutrients and is a superb supplement to any diet but it only comprises of cannabinoids in very small amounts, as it is made from the seeds of the hemp plant. The oil is derived by grinding or pressing the seeds at a low temperature of 120°F and it maintains its nutritional value and flavour.

Although hemp seed oil is not a nutritional supplement, it can be added to CBD supplements as basis for these products. Extracts of CBD oil is inclined to getting thicker making it difficult to administer. Combining them into hemp oil can settle this problem.

Cold pressing is a very good method for getting hemp seed oil, however it does not come in handy for the production of CBD oil as the oil is derived from the plants stems and stalks.

2. The Rick Simpson's technique for cannabis oil

This method of CBD oil extraction uses naphtha or petroleum as solvents. The Rick's technique, although effective in obtaining the compounds which are active from the cannabis plant, it usually results to getting terpenes and CBD in lower concentration and a higher concentration of THC.

It can therefore be said, that this is not the best choice if you are looking at obtaining a rich CBD Oil. It is also considered not to be safe due to the remnants that may be left from the solvents which may inhibit the functions of the immune system.

3. Extracting with olive or ethanol

Olive oil and Ethanol can be used for taking out cannabinoids and terpenes from the cannabis plant in full range and they possess the advantage of being secured for consumption too.

Ethanol extracts chlorophyll which makes the final product to have an unpleasant taste and a not-so fascinating colour. This chlorophyll can be removed by filtrating the extract but this extra step will cause a significant amount of the CBD to be removed.

Olive oil is a substitute but it also has its setbacks. The positive side of taking out the cannabinoids with olive oil is that the method is easy and only requires heating up the oil to 200°F and filtrating the extract. Sadly, this extract cannot be condensed. Although it contains CBD, you would need to ingest large proportion of CBD oil extracted this way to see significant health effects.

4. The Super critical CO2 extraction

This is a non-toxic and exceptionally efficient technique to get CBD oil but it's more expensive. It needs expertise and complex equipment. This method uses secure solvents and guarantees extracts which are highly pure and potent.

The oil obtained through this process is a complete range of cannabinoid-rich product containing numerous health advantages. The oil has a light - yellow colour and transparent.   The oil obtained is superior to extracts obtained from previously stated techniques.

Chapter 4

Is CBD oil safe to Use?

Many that are curious about beginning with CBD oil do worry about the safety of using this product. They usually want to know if it will get high and if it's safe to use around kids.

Thankfully, CBD does not cause harm because it is non-psychoactive and has minimal side effects.

CBD is non-toxic

CBD is considered safe to use and non-toxic for humans even at high amounts.

A research carried out in the Department of Clinical, Toxicological and Food Sciences Analysis at the University of Sao Paulo, Brazil explored the safety and effects of cannabidiol.

This study suggested that the administration of CBD is safe to use and non-poisonous to humans and animals.

CBD Oil is Non-Psychoactive

CBD oil contains only trace levels of THC and it is therefore considered safe for use by you and even your entire family without fear of intoxication.

Side Effects of CBD

Although CBD is safe to use, it has some few side effects which you should consider before embarking on its use. The Known side effects of CBD are:

1. Dry mouth

The commonly described side effect of the administration of CBD is the dry sensation it causes within the mouth. This appears to be caused by the connection of the endocannabinoid system in inhibiting saliva secretion. This effect may be mitigated by drinking a glass of water.

2. Drowsiness or Wakefulness

CBD can cause drowsiness when high dose is consumed. If this is the way you feel when you ingest CBD, it is safe not to drive a vehicle or operate any machine equipment.

In most cases however, CBD serves as a wake-inducing agent.

3. Low Blood pressure

High dosage of CBD oil daily may cause a minimum drop in blood pressure. This drop in blood pressure is often connected with feelings of light-headedness. This side effect is temporary and can be mitigated by drinking a cup of tea or coffee.

4. Increased quiver in Parkinson's disease when high dose CBD is consumed.

Research carried out by some group of scientists confirms that high doses of CBD may worsen muscle movement in individuals that suffers from Parkinson's disease. Other studies also recommend cannabidiol to be safe and well tolerable by patients of Parkinson's disease.

In this case, reducing CBD dose intake will reduce this possible side effect. Sufferers of Parkinson's disease should consult with their doctor before consuming CBD and should start by taking smaller doses.

5. Inhibition of hepatic drug metabolism

CBD can interact with specific series of pharmaceutical drugs because it has been proven to inhibit cytochrome p450, a group of liver enzymes responsible for the breaking down of an extensive range of pharmaceutical medicines. If a high dose of CBD is ingested, the cannabinoid can temporarily neutralize the activity of p450 enzymes, thus changing the way drugs are metabolized inside the body. The effect is however minor.

If you're currently using pharmaceutical drugs and still interested in consuming CBD, discuss with your doctor or pharmacist.

How does Cannabidiol (CBD) work inside one's body?

CBD is the core active ingredient in hemp and unlike Tetrahydrocannabinol (THC), it is not psychoactive, therefore, it does not get a person intoxicated. The body system of human comprises of endocannabinoid system and receptors spread through the body and brain. THC triggers two receptors (CB1 and CB2), while CBD does not exactly stimulate any of these receptors; it rather stimulates other receptors like adenosine, serotonin receptors and vanilloid.

Chapter 5

How to buy CBD Oil Online

Tips and Tricks of purchasing high quality CBD Oil

CBD oil is an enchanting natural remedy that originates from the Cannabis plant. The oil functions as a herbal remedy for many medical sicknesses devoid of any psychoactive consequences.

It permits a person to keep healthy and maintain a stable state. It keeps the body safe from undesirable side effects of pharmaceutical medicines.

Getting the original CBD oil could be very discouraging especially if you are new to CBD oil. Buyers have several techniques to purchasing CBD. You can either purchase CBD oil from dispensaries, online stores, natural herbalists, and co-ops.

The CBD oil is bought depending on the accessibility, preferred ways of consumption and means of applications such as tinctures, CBD oil, infused edibles, vaporizers, vape pens, topical, or as transdermal patches.

Buyers ask many questions during the purchase of CBD oil. They want to know if purchasing the oil is legal in the state they reside in or not. The answer depends on the method of extraction.

If CBD oil is hauled out from the hemp plant, then it is completely lawful devoid of psychoactive consequences.

There are guidelines and tricks of purchasing the oil online if you are using it as an effective and secure alternative treatment for health related problems.

This reason is due to the fact that the CBD industry is not properly controlled due to the poor quality products that are promptly available in the market stores along with the CBD oils which cause psychoactive consequences due to presence of the high THC content.

How do I buy the CBD Oil?

The CBD oil is generally available in recent times due to the constant research and studies which have proved its efficacy. It is now made legal in the world because of its non-psychoactive effects, though, it can be a daunting task to get reliable CBD product.

You are to pay adequate attention when searching for quality CBD products so as to purchase the original CBD product.

Many people mix up CBD oil for THC (the ingredient found in cannabis which is responsible for the psychoactive effects that leads to having a high feeling and this has resulted into different mixed opinions and reviews about the CBD product. Many people still perceive CBD oil to be a drug that provides a high feeling effect due to its association with cannabis. However, laboratory and clinical tests has proven that CBD oil can't and will not get the user intoxicated.

Great Tips and Tricks to buy CBD oil

These are the simple steps you need to consider to get a high quality and rich CBD oil from online stores. Reliable and trustworthy sellers keeps their integrity by always providing you with detailed information connected to the product you are purchasing.

1.   Search for first-class products rather than the reduced-priced products.

Once you have made the decision to buy CBD oil, go to Google where you will find numerous search results. There are different products readily available in the market place due to the difference in price, extraction methods and quantity.

Keep in mind that getting quality CBD oil can never be low-prices and that is a fact. Many people have chosen low prices over quality and leave negative reviews when the aim of purchasing the CBD oil is not achieved. Bear in mind that if you are aim at getting inexpensive products from the market, it can never be effective.

Many providers of CBD oil and sellers have capitalized on the point that CBD oil is gradually gaining popularity all over the globe due to its health benefit and have decided to profit easily by selling fake products of CBD. Be wise; don't be lured by low prices.

The best way to recognize a high quality CBD product is to request for third-party lab inquiry from the vendor.

Authentic CBD oil providers will feed you with basic information about the product as well as the source and full concentration of cannabidiol.

Check to see the concentration of cannabidiol because the greater the cannabidiol level, the more effective the product will be.

2.   CBD volume

Check the CBD volume within the product when buying CBD oil. Since the CBD oils are obtainable in different volumes, you would need to know the quantity of CBD you will be ingesting for every dose taken.

You cannot afford to go on an overdose as you will need to know the amount of CBD oil your body can carry to cure the medical condition.

The CBD oil concentration relies on the fundamental health issues. Therefore, it is best you consult with someone who has used CBD oil already or you strictly adhere to the dosage guide. It is also advisable you begin with a low dose of CBD oil and increase gradually.

3. Volume of hemp seed oil

There are two main components you should be concerned about when you are about to buy the CBD oil.

a. CBD volume

b. Volume of hemp seed oil

The Hemp seed oil volume is the quantity of hemp oil available in the product.

Hemp oil also has its health benefit but you need to be sure of the CBD concentration in the product you are purchasing when buying CBD products. Buying an item with high concentration of hemp oil and a low content of CBD is like taking in fish oil with additional EPA and DHA without the main ingredients.

4. Study the CBD product Label

Some hemp products are sold with psychoactive compounds which results in unpleasant effects. However, the CBD oil is extracted from industrial hemp or food-grade hemp with little or no amount of THC.

So, choose only CBD products with non-psychoactive ingredients as stated on the labels.

5. CBD concentration

The concentration of CBD is all about the amount of CBD present in the whole volume of CBD product. As earlier stated, CBD oil has several other products aside from CBD so bear in mind the amount of CBD present before buying any CBD product.

The permitted dosage for starters is between 2-3gms. However, you can begin with 10 mg depending on your height and weight and adjust accordingly.

To achieve the desired result of this oil, use the product consistently. If you are unable to achieve the desired effect with first dosage, increase your consumption of CBD and observe the result over time.

6. Check the product website for product reviews

The CBD oil industry is still fresh and young. Getting a company with proven track records about the CBD products can be very tough.

When buying your quality CBD products, make sure you are buying products from a vendor of good repute by reading the product reviews on the internet.

7. Customer service

The integrity of the vendors can be quickly accessed by contacting them directly. Reliable and well recognised companies have a good customer service representative that answers all queries concerning a particular purchase.

You can easily get in touch with them via phone, email or live chat. The customer service representative would be glad to provide the answers to all your queries.

8. Manufacturers Identification of where the plant was originated from

The CBD oil can be identified by examining the product to be free from chemical pesticides and herbicides.

The CBD plant should be cultivated on a land where there is no prior refuse dump as the plants can take in contaminants and industrial wastes. These wastes can be deposited into the body once CBD is consumed.

9. Method of Extraction

The procedures of CBD oil extraction have the capacity to cause creation of harmful solvents in traces.

Dependable CBD manufacturers choose an extraction technique that gives the purest type of the CBD oil.

The well known method of extraction used by recognized companies is the Supercritical Fluid Extraction using Carbon dioxide or CO2 technology.

10.   Go for a non - GMO product

Genetically modified organism (GMO) is a modern technology and not much is identified about its effect on the human body. Scientific studies have however reported that GMO's contain toxins, boosts the susceptibility of disease, less nutritious, and might damage the soil which will call for increased application of pesticides.

In conclusion, CBD oil industries are daily growing and many industrialists are getting into this line to assist the patients who are faced with underlying medical problems.

However, as a buyer, you need to be more careful so as not to buy fake CBD oil. Don't be carried away by the low prices. Get high quality oil and your recovery would

be faster than you ever imagined.

Chapter 6

Simple Hemp Oil Recipes

Hemp seeds & Roasted Avocado Toast

A Tasty Toast!

Ingredients:

Sourdough bread, sliced (4)

1-2 Garlic bulbs, roasted & cloves removed

1 large sized avocado, sliced thinly or puree

Hemp Hearts

Red pepper, crushed

Pepper

Salt

Directions:

1. Toast the bread.

2. Smudge the sliced bread with the roasted garlic.

3. Arrange the sliced or pureed avocado on the bread.

4. Now, sprinkle bread with preferred quantity of crushed pepper (chilli flakes), hemp seeds, pepper and salt.

Hemp Seed Humus

A tasty vegan recipe, low in carbs and healthy in fats!

Ingredients:

4 tablespoon hemp seeds

3 cups chickpeas, canned or cooked

4 teaspoon lemon juice

2 small garlic cloves, minced

2 tablespoon water

6 tablespoon olive oil

Red pepper flakes, paprika and chopped parsley (for garnish)

1 teaspoon salt

Directions:

1. Crush the hemp seeds in a grinder.

2. Put the grinded hemp seeds inside a food processor.

3. Add lemon juice, chickpeas, oil, minced garlic, and salt.

4. Blend all for a minute or until soft. Add more water as desired to get thinner hummus.

5. Serve and drizzle with some oil, red pepper, paprika and parsley.

Almond Butter Hemp Seed Banana Sushi

Ridiculously simple and tasty!

Ingredients:

1 medium banana

1 tablespoon almond butter

1 teaspoon hemp seeds

Directions:

1. Peel the banana.

2. Spread the butter on the banana, ensure you coat both sides.

3. Sprinkle the hemp hearts.

4. Put the banana in the freezer for a minimum of one hour.

5. Slice the banana about an inch thick, just like sushi, serve.

Blackberry Pomegranate & Hemp Protein Chia Pudding

A Dairy-free, Gluten-Free & Paleo Friendly!

Ingredients:

Chia Pudding:

1 tablespoon organic sweetener

1 cup almond milk

1 tablespoon organic chia seeds

1 tablespoon Blackberry Pomegranate Hemp Protein

For the Topping

1/2 cup organic pomegranate seeds

1/2 cup organic blackberries

Directions:

1. In a mason jar, add all chia pudding ingredients. Seal the jar tightly and shake well until all ingredients are blended together.

2. Refrigerate the jar for 30 minutes to 1 hour, or until the pudding firms up.

3. Remove the jar from the refrigerator; add the organic blackberries and the pomegranate seeds to the top.

Almond, Dates, Coconut & Banana Smoothie with Hemp seed

The list of hemp seed recipes will be incomplete without a smoothie!

Ingredients:

1 big banana, frozen

2 tablespoon hemp seeds, hulled

One-quarter teaspoon cinnamon

1 cup coconut milk, full-fat

4 dates, fresh & pitted

Almonds, crushed for serving

Hemps seeds (for serving)

Directions:

1. Combine all ingredients in a blender, blend till smooth.

2. Add more spices if needed.

3. Pour into glass cups, top with almonds and the hemp seeds.

4. Serve.

THE END

Did you enjoy reading this book? Please check out other books recommended by the author.

About The Author

Hirsch Friedrich Pebble was born and raised in New York. He is a creative writer with many books to his credit.

He started his writing career as a freelance writer and came across CBD and hemp oil in one of his writings. His quest for knowledge made him study further and having used it, knows the importance of the rich CBD hemp oil.

He loves to grow plants in his garden. He is blessed with a wonderful family and he is an accomplished motivational speaker in his home town.

Disclaimer

This book contains information that is intended to help the readers be better informed consumers of health care.

It is presented as general advice on health care.

This book is not intended to be a substitute for the medical advice of a licensed physician. The reader should consult with their doctor in any matters relating to his/her health.

Recommendations

http://getbook.at/cookbooklowcarb

http://getbook.at/cookbook

http://getbook.at/ketogenic-diet

http://getbook.at/aboutcats

http://getbook.at/transgendgerworld

http://getbook.at/cookbooklowcarb

Acknowledgement

To God and my inestimable clients who made me see the need to study more on CBD for the treatment of my diabetes.

I appreciate you all.